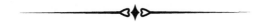

DISCLAIMER AND/OR LEGAL NOTICES:

The information presented herein represents the view of the author as of the date of publication. Because of the rate with which conditions change, the author reserves the right to alter and update their opinion based on the new conditions. The material is for educational purposes only. While every attempt has been made to verify the information provided in this journal, neither the author nor their affiliates/partners assume any responsibility for errors, inaccuracies or omissions. Any slights of people or organisations are unintentional. If advice concerning legal or related matters is needed, the services of a fully qualified professional should be sought. This journal is not intended for use as a source of legal or medical advice. Any reference to any person or business whether living or dead is purely coincidental.

I dedicate this journal to Neha Narne: my beloved teenage Mentee and friend who is bright, intelligently gifted, caring, generous, compassionate as well as beautiful inside and out.

May you always remain curious about life and people, Neha!

TABLE OF CONTENTS

INTRODUCTION

How are you?

In your lifetime you're probably going to be asked this a few thousand times. Or at least it seems like you are. The problem is, when a question becomes so common it tends to carry less meaning. We answer, "Fine" without thinking, an automatic response much like saying "Hello."

But are you fine?   Really?

All too often we're busy. Stressed. There's just too much going on in the day and we're already short on time. We're not as fine as we like to pretend, we are. If we're honest, we're probably not spending as much time on ourselves as we ought to. In short, we're neglecting self-care.

If you think self-care isn't a big deal, then consider these statistics taken from various studies all over the world:

- Approximately 75% of people are chronically dehydrated.
- Approximately 39% of adults are overweight.
- Sleepless cities revealed as one in three adults suffer from insomnia
- Approximately 69% of Employees, Many in Safety-critical Jobs, are Tired at Work.
- Approximately 18% of adults are anxious.
- Approximately 5% of adults are depressed.

If you just winced from reading this list, you're not alone. No, none of us is fine, and it is time we did something about it.

In this book, we will go through the following:

- Take care of your wellbeing including mental health.
- This book gives structure to the year; however, you may start with any month.
- The book provides unique exercises.
- Self-Reflection Questions.

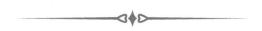

I'm going to explore the importance of self-care. More importantly, I'm going to show you how to build new habits which will help you practice better self-care. How? Well, you're going to want to keep this book handy, because you and I are going to explore a new self-care strategy every month. By this time next year, you're going to feel like an entirely different person.

So, get ready to dig in. It's going to be an exciting new year leading to an exciting new you!

WHAT IS SELF CARE ?

According to Kelly Donahue, self-care can be best described as *"Any thought or action that we do deliberately to take care of our mental, spiritual, emotional, and physical health. Self-care is doing and thinking the things that serve our highest good and help to create the best version of us."*

So it is clear from this definition that self-care goes deeper than spa days, etc. It is important, therefore, to recognise that self-care is a journey and as such if you fall off track get back on the bike as soon as you can, get going again and do so with the same kindness towards yourself as you would show your loved ones. Consider and write your journal within this wider and deeper context.

WHY SELF CARE ?

Why is it so hard to take care of ourselves? The answer could be found in our own compassion. We spend so much time worrying about those who we love and making sure we meet our responsibilities; we forget about a very basic truth.

We cannot fully take care of anyone else, unless we are in a position to do so. Most people these days fly and you will be aware that on planes the flight safety instructions given state very clearly that individuals must put on their own oxygen masks first, before helping anybody else put on theirs.

WHAT DOES THIS MEAN?
Think about these basic signs and symptoms of what happens when self-care suffers:

- You have a harder time thinking.
- You're sick more often.
- Your quality of work suffers.
- You feel overwhelmed.
- You wake up tired, even after a full night of sleep.
- You forget what you're about to say.
- You miss deadlines.
- You find yourself isolating and avoiding social situations.
- You're cranky or feel "off."
- You snap at people.
- Simple tasks seem to take a lot of effort.
- You forget little things, such as returning library books.
- You're dragging yourself through the day.
- Decisions become really difficult, even simple ones.
- You're worried or anxious though you're not sure why.
- You can't sit still.
- You're not eating right, either too much or too little.
- You're not following through on promises.
- You're ignoring things you used to enjoy, either through lack of interest or energy.
- You've lost enthusiasm.

Now think about what this means when it comes to taking care of others. How in the world are you supposed to take care of any outside responsibilities, even ones you love such as taking care of your kids, when you're feeling like that?

It doesn't really work, does it?

Worse, we're not doing what's right by the one person who's supposed to matter more than anything. YOU!

The "Selfishness" of Self-Care for Women?

Perhaps the biggest thing to get in the way of self-care though, is the nagging feeling we're not supposed to be spending so much time on ourselves. After all, isn't it pretty self-centered to be worrying about yourself?

Not so. Writer and activist Parker Palmer perhaps put it best:

Self-care is never a selfish act - it is simply good stewardship of the only gift I have, the gift I was put on earth to offer others. Anytime we can listen to our true self and give the care it requires, we do it not only for ourselves, but for the many others whose lives we touch.

In short, only when we're truly at our best, do we have the ability to give to those around us. Our best work is made possible by good health and a keen intellect. It's here where we do our best work. There isn't a responsibility in the world which can be met if you don't have the health and ability to do the work.

Still struggling with the idea of self-care? Then consider this last very important point. Self-care is what keeps you around to make sure you get stuff done. Without self-care, our work suffers. So do we.

Without proper self-care it can be argued you're taking years off your life.

Maybe self-care doesn't quite sound so selfish anymore when put in those terms.

10

What Self-Care Could Do for YOU!

As you read through this next section, I want you to think about what you're reading. Imagine the year being laid out for you. See how the changes come together to form a picture of a new, and rather different you, one that experiences life a little differently than what we saw listed at the beginning of the chapter.

With good mental and physical health, you will:

- ...have no trouble thinking.
- ...never have a sick day.
- ...do your best work every single day.
- ...can't wait to start the day.
- ...look forward to what comes next with enthusiasm.
- ...be articulate and well-spoken.
- ...never miss a deadline.
- ...enjoy a great social life.
- ...be in a great mood.

- ...be patient with those around you.
- ...handle complex tasks with ease.
- ...be on top of things.
- ...feel like you can keep going all day long.
- ...have no trouble making decisions.
- ...be relaxed and calm.
- ...look and feel great.
- ...follow up in a timely manner.
- ...always have something going on.
- ...be full of enthusiasm, every single day.

Sound pretty good?

Then what are you waiting for?

2022

The Year You Regain Your Youthful Vibrancy

When trying to build a habit of self-care, the whole process can seem pretty daunting. There are so many different areas you will need to focus in order to be truly healthy and happy. This is why it's so important to start small. Studies have shown "baby steps" work best when it comes to forming new habits. It's for this reason this book is laid out in a way to keep you from becoming overwhelmed by new material.

From here on out, you're going to focus only on one habit at a time. Each habit is meant to be formed over the course of one month. Do not work ahead, or think you can form all 12 habits in just one month. Doing so is a sure recipe for disaster. The key here is to stick to slow and steady progress. This is where we will create the most lasting change. Think of it as running a marathon instead of sprinting a short distance.

The following is a list of the habits you will be focusing on:

1. Sleep.

2. Eating Right.

3. Exercise.

4. Practice Gratitude.

5. Treat Yourself.

6. Setting Healthy Boundaries.

7. Go Outside.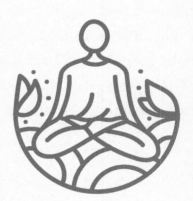

8. Learn Something New.

9. Relax and De-stress.

10. Work on Relationships.

11. Be More Mindful.

12. Reflect.

Life is a Personal Journey!

When we're on a personal journey, we often don't even tell those around us about our goals or share them with only a select few. This tends to mean we likewise keep much of the journey to ourselves. The tips in this guided journal work best with these kinds of journeys.

Examples of personal journeys include (but are not limited to):

- Losing Weight
- Erasing Procrastination
- Improving Self-Talk
- Better Attention to Self-Care
- Higher Quality of Sleep
- Eating Better

Of all the journeys we take, the personal ones seem to be the ones that encourage the most self-reflection. By keeping a journal, you have a record of your thoughts and feelings as you explore the changes you're experiencing. Because what you're doing is so personal, this journal also becomes a record of progress and a way to enjoy again every milestone you experience.

SHARE WHAT YOU'RE DOING

Even if your journey feels very private, having someone to share it with makes it that much more enjoyable. Enlist someone you are especially close to who will act as support. The perfect person is one you can both laugh and cry with, so pick someone who is equal parts cheerleader and shoulder to cry on.

If you can't find this particular person, maybe you need to enlist more than one person to play each role. What makes this even nicer is how much closer you'll feel to this friend(s) as this kind of sharing builds a more intimate and special relationship between you.

CELEBRATE OFTEN

Milestones can be especially important in personal journeys as they mark a special kind of progress in becoming a better person. So, make sure you take time to celebrate every one of them in some small way that makes you feel fantastic. Be sure to choose rewards that won't impede your progress.

For example, the last thing you need is chocolate as a reward for losing weight. A brand new to you item to wear (thrift shops can help you stay on a budget) or even a special bubble bath can be just the thing, though.

HOW TO USE THIS JOURNAL

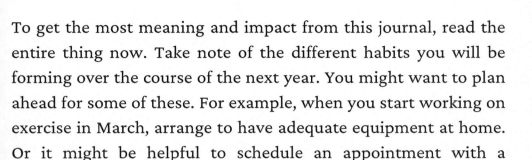

To get the most meaning and impact from this journal, read the entire thing now. Take note of the different habits you will be forming over the course of the next year. You might want to plan ahead for some of these. For example, when you start working on exercise in March, arrange to have adequate equipment at home. Or it might be helpful to schedule an appointment with a nutritionist/health coach to talk about nutrition before February.

As you focus on the month you are currently in, read through the various tips and choose the ones which you think will be most helpful. These will be the habits you are focusing on building through this month.

Keep in mind you will be performing these habits on a daily basis, so you might want to write them down or keep them somewhere handy to remind yourself of what you're doing.

Remember, we form new habits best through repetition. The more often you practice these tips, the more likely they are to become part of your daily routine.

Sounds pretty simple ? Let's get started !

JANUARY: SLEEP

Are you one of the women included in the 80% of people experiencing insomnia?

How sleep-deprived are you? If you're like most people, you probably are. In fact, 3/4 of people polled admit they're too tired to work. It's pretty safe to assume, this isn't caused by boredom or even the physicality of their jobs. Especially when you add to this statistic the fact that 80% of people feel like they don't get enough to sleep at least a couple of times a month, and 11% of people have chronic sleep problems which keep them from getting enough rest.

Phew, that's a lot of tired people!
How do you go about fixing your sleep schedule where so many people have failed? You start during the day, long before you go to bed.

Get Into the Light.
We all need natural light. Our bodies have a natural circadian rhythm which dictates when we sleep and when we wake. If we never see the sun, we don't know where we are in the day. Spending at least two hours a day where we can see natural light becomes very important in keeping your body rhythms in check.

Drop the Naps.
Daytime naps can do more harm than good. Unless you're really exhausted and need to catch a few zzzs, you'd do better to adjust your schedule to where you go to bed earlier than to nap now.

No Caffeine.

Well, you can still have your morning coffee, but once you hit afternoon you'll sleep better if you quit drinking anything with caffeine.

Forget the Blues.

Forget the blue light in the evening completely. Sadly, this is the kind of light which comes off of just about everything with a screen you can imagine. While this might seem kind of arbitrary, keep this important fact in mind: blue light makes your body think it's still daytime. The longer you stay in front of a screen, the surer your body will make you need to be awake. By putting the screens away, a couple of hours before bedtime, you're letting your body know it's time for sleep.

Follow a Bedtime Routine.

In fact, the more routine your evening is, the easier it is to fall asleep. Dim the lights, and do quiet things in the half hour before bed. No more exercise, no more TV. This signals your body to what comes next.

Create the Atmosphere.

Your bedroom should be dark and cosy. The right temperature should be a little bit cooler in the room than if you were up and about. Make sure your mattress is firm and is replaced often enough to provide good support. Likewise, you're going to want to replace your pillows often as well – every one to two years is best.

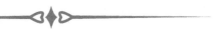

HAVING TROUBLE SLEEPING?

If you're not falling asleep you might need to try a few of these pro-tips:

Get Up.

If you're still not asleep after half an hour, get up and move around. Do something such as read or complete whatever small task might be nagging at you.

Do so in dim lights, without looking at the clock. Return to bed when you start feeling tired. It's better to get up and move around than lay staring at the ceiling half the night.

Try to Relax.

There are various meditation routines or exercises which can help you get to sleep. Try tensing and relaxing each muscle group, slowly, in turn. Or listen to a guided visualisation to help guide you toward sleep.

Adjust Your Bedtime (and Wake Time)

We all sleep better on a routine. By going to bed at the same time every single night and getting up at the same time every day we tend to fall asleep much faster.

Note: If insomnia is a frequent problem, you might want to keep a sleep diary for a week or two and take it to your doctor. It never hurts to have an expert weigh in.

Please write notes of your thoughts about your relationship
with sleep during this month. Choose an Adjective or a Phrase to describe
how you feel about sleep each day.

WEEK 1

- Monday

  _____

  _____

- Tuesday

  _____

  _____

- Wednesday

  _____

  _____

- Thursday

  _____

  _____

- Friday

  _____

  _____

- Saturday

  _____

  _____

- Sunday

  _____

  _____

WEEK 2

- Monday

  _____

  _____

- Tuesday

  _____

  _____

- Wednesday

  _____

  _____

- Thursday

  _____

  _____

- Friday

  _____

  _____

- Saturday

  _____

  _____

- Sunday

  _____

  _____

WEEK 3

- Monday

  _____

  _____

- Tuesday

  _____

  _____

- Wednesday

  _____

  _____

- Thursday

  _____

  _____

- Friday

  _____

  _____

- Saturday

  _____

  _____

- Sunday

  _____

  _____

WEEK 4

- Monday

  _____

  _____

- Tuesday

  _____

  _____

- Wednesday

  _____

  _____

- Thursday

  _____

  _____

- Friday

  _____

  _____

- Saturday

  _____

  _____

- Sunday

  _____

  _____

FEBRUARY: EATING RIGHT

Drink. More. Water! Don't Eat Your Feelings!

Eating right can mean so many things to different people. What you might not realise, is there is more than one way to eat correctly. With so much worry as to which diet is best such as vegetarian, keto, paleo, and others, the most common reason people don't eat well is they don't know where to begin. You should start with your doctor.

If you have underlying medical conditions, or food allergies, the proper diet will be whatever your doctor tells you it should be. After all, following a diet which includes a lot of dairy when you're allergic to milk is only going to make you miserable. Once you have this guidance, it's time to get into the nitty gritty of following the diet which is best for you.

The Universal Truths.
There are some tips which are universal regardless of what your core diet is. These are the habits we're going to focus on. The rest will have to be up to you. If you're going vegan, you'll have to research how to do so in a healthy way. The same goes for any other dietary consideration. Here's what we do know:

Hydrate.
When the statistics show 75% of people are dehydrated at any given moment, the answer should be obvious. DRINK. MORE. WATER!

In fact, the rule of thumb is to drink half an ounce of water for every pound you weigh in the course of a day. So, if you weigh 150 pounds, you should be drinking 75 ounces of water. Yikes! No wonder we don't drink enough!

Keep in mind though, some foods are rich in liquid, so you can get some of your hydration by eating fresh fruits and even vegetables.

Focus on Whole Foods.
The definition of whole foods is "plant foods which are unprocessed and unrefined, or processed and refined as little as possible, before being consumed." (Wikipedia). In other words, fresh foods are always best. For some great options, try visiting a farmer's market to explore what's local and seasonal.

Drop Processed Foods.
Processed food is always going to be the enemy no matter what diet you're following. Things which are processed are full of sugars, trans fats, and salt which you really don't need. Also, it's more expensive to eat the processed stuff, so avoiding it isn't only good for you, it's good for your bank account.

Limit Sugar.
If you're diabetic, this is a must. Even if you're not, there's no true benefit to refined sugar, especially when it's presented in sweets. If you're craving dessert, you'd be better off with a piece of fruit.

Meal Times.
We process food better when we eat at regular times every day. Skipping meals only hurts you in the long run, and also causes you to overeat when you do eat later on.

Eat More Often.

Your body processes food better when you're not stuffing yourself at every meal. Rather than having three big meals every day, consider six very small meals spaced out over time.

Re-organise Your Cupboards

If you find yourself eating while watching TV, or for energy throughout the day, it's really better if you don't buy the bad stuff at all. Keeping it out of the kitchen and replacing it with healthier alternatives will keep you snacking, but in a better way. How about some veggies and dip instead of those chips?

Process Your Feelings.

Finally, it's very common for people to eat as a way of dealing with depression, anxiety, or worry. Rather than grabbing something to eat, why not journal what's going on? What are you feeling right now? What trigger are you responding to? By acknowledging your emotions and working through them, you'll find the cravings for food will be less strong.

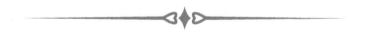

In the end, if you're still struggling with the food issues, don't be afraid to talk to someone about how you're feeling. There are some great groups such as Overeater's Anonymous and professional counselors who specialise in food issues who will help you to work through bad food habits and help you get back on track.

Please write notes of your thoughts about your relationship with food during this month. Choose an Adjective or a Phrase to describe how you feel about food each day.

WEEK 1

- Monday

  _____

  _____

- Tuesday

  _____

  _____

- Wednesday

  _____

  _____

- Thursday

  _____

  _____

- Friday

  _____

  _____

- Saturday

  _____

  _____

- Sunday

  _____

  _____

WEEK 2

- Monday

  _____

  _____

- Tuesday

  _____

  _____

- Wednesday

  _____

  _____

- Thursday

  _____

  _____

- Friday

  _____

  _____

- Saturday

  _____

  _____

- Sunday

  _____

  _____

WEEK 3

- Monday

  _____

  _____

- Tuesday

  _____

  _____

- Wednesday

  _____

  _____

- Thursday

  _____

  _____

- Friday

  _____

  _____

- Saturday

  _____

  _____

- Sunday

  _____

  _____

WEEK 4

Monday

_____

_____

Tuesday

_____

_____

Wednesday

_____

_____

Thursday

_____

_____

Friday

_____

_____

Saturday

_____

_____

Sunday

_____

_____

MARCH: EXERCISE.

The human body is created for movement. How much do you move yours?   What do you think about exercise and how much is part of your routine?

Exercise is probably one of those things which has already made you personal self-care list in the past. If so, you're not alone. Every yea 59% of people put personal fitness on their list of New Year': Resolutions.

Here again, a talk with your doctor is absolutely necessary before getting started. You're going to want to work with their approval especially before you go all out and start practicing for a triathlon.
Once you have, it's time to get started. Again, there are a lot of ways to exercise, each one tailored to your personal likes and interests. There is no one way which is right. The important thing is to do something which you like, because you're going to be exercising often. If you start off thinking this is drudgery, it's going to be.

From there, what steps should you follow?

Get an Assessment.
You're going to need to be very honest about what you're capable of doing. If you've been a couch potato for a while, the last thing you should even attempt would be to swim twenty laps a day or run five miles. There are some places online which can help you figure out your fitness level. Your better bet if you can afford it? Book a session with a personal trainer and get their assessment. It's going to be a lot more accurate, and they'll be able to help you set up a workout regimen which will work for you.

Create a Goal.

What does being fit and healthy look like to you? If you're aiming for weight loss, you might want to find a chart online to give you some guidance for what's healthy for you and use that as a general guideline. Then create some steps to reach this goal. Remember to start small. You shouldn't be losing more than 2 pounds a week. For fitness goals, you'll want to start with where you are now and work up gradually to where you'd like to be. So, if you want to be able to run a 5k, you might start with being able to walk 1k and work up from there as you're comfortable doing.

Create Your Daily Routine.

Once you have a goal, break it down into little pieces. Exercise should happen daily, so put it on your schedule right now before you forget. Give yourself enough time without rushing and keep in mind you're starting small and building up. So while 15 minutes a day might be good right now, by the end of the month you might want to allow yourself 30 minutes a day or more. Building this much time into your schedule now will help to assure you can expand on what you're doing easily without 'falling off the wagon' due to lack of time.

Mix it Up.

To keep from getting bored, you might want to create more than one workout routine. How about working abs on one day and doing aerobic exercise the next? It's actually healthier to work this way, too!

Chart Your Progress – and Reward Yourself Often.

Keeping track of what you're doing means you're more likely to keep it up. Especially if you make it fun by giving yourself little prizes for making it to a certain milestone. (No food prizes though. How about a movie instead?)

Check in.

How are you doing? You're going to want to assess yourself often. Pay attention to injuries or other problems as they come up and be sure to talk to your doctor if anything seems serious. If things are going well and you're making your workout goals too easily, it might be time to up your game.

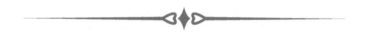

A final word? For the best results, don't exercise alone. A workout partner adds accountability and just makes the whole idea a lot more fun. Good luck!

Please write notes of your thoughts about exercise/movement during this month. Choose an Adjective or a Phrase to describe how you feel about exercise/movement each day.

WEEK 1

- Monday

  _____

  _____

- Tuesday

  _____

  _____

- Wednesday

  _____

  _____

- Thursday

  _____

  _____

- Friday

  _____

  _____

- Saturday

  _____

  _____

- Sunday

  _____

  _____

WEEK 2

- Monday

  _____

  _____

- Tuesday

  _____

  _____

- Wednesday

  _____

  _____

- Thursday

  _____

  _____

- Friday

  _____

  _____

- Saturday

  _____

  _____

- Sunday

  _____

  _____

WEEK 3

Monday

_____

_____

Tuesday

_____

_____

Wednesday

_____

_____

Thursday

_____

_____

Friday

_____

_____

Saturday

_____

_____

Sunday

_____

_____

WEEK 4

- Monday

  _____

  _____

- Tuesday

  _____

  _____

- Wednesday

  _____

  _____

- Thursday

  _____

  _____

- Friday

  _____

  _____

- Saturday

  _____

  _____

- Sunday

  _____

  _____

APRIL: PRACTICE GRATITUDE

What are your views about gratitude? How do you practice gratitude? Do you express gratitude and how do you do this?

It's so important to your mental well-being to be grateful for what you already have. What you might not realise is just how much gratitude really is self-care.

Without gratitude in our lives, we start to fall into a cycle of negativity. We see the world as bleak and without hope. We might even start thinking there isn't much to celebrate about mankind. After all, the news is full of people behaving their worst.

With gratitude, these thought processes start to shift around. When we're able to be thankful for the things we have, we also gain satisfaction in these items. We start yearning less for what's out of reach. Dissatisfaction falls. Better yet, when we're thankful for the people in our lives, we start seeing humanity itself in a better life. The world isn't so dark. We realise people are better than we give them credit for.

How do you practice gratitude? Try these tips:

Start a Gratitude Journal.
What are you thankful for? Sometimes it can be hard to come up with these items. We don't always notice what we're grateful for. By writing them down as they occur to us, we have a record we can refer back to when we need it. Pro-tip? Write in your Gratitude Journal every night before bed. You can record the things which happened during the day for which you are thankful.

This puts you in a good headspace as you prepare to sleep, and will make for a better night.

Say It Often.
Have you ever had a moment where you just felt grateful? Whenever this emotion comes up, say out loud what you're thankful for. Doing this on a regular basis changes the conversation both in your head, and with those around you.

Write a Note.
Who are you grateful for? What kind acts have you appreciated? The old standby of writing thank you notes might feel like they've gone the way of the dinosaur, but anyone who has ever received such a note will tell you how good they felt when they got one. Who can you write to today, to express your thanks?

Couple Gratitude with the Mundane.
Doing chores? Think thankful thoughts as you fold laundry or empty the dishwasher. Looking for the positive while doing something which normally doesn't stir those emotions will make the whole day feel brighter.

Grab Some Affirmations.
Having trouble with thinking grateful thoughts? Write down some quotes on gratitude or other positive affirmations having to do with being thankful and scatter them everywhere to help you get into a grateful mindset.

Make it a Group Activity.
At Thanksgiving it's not uncommon for people to go around the table and say what they're grateful for before they eat.

Make this a regular practice at the family dinner table. Ask your friends what they're grateful for the next time you're out. Want to take it to the next level? Create a gratitude luncheon with your friends where the goal is for everyone to talk about something they're grateful for.

Volunteer.
You really loved it when someone else lent a hand in your life. Do the same for someone else. This is gratitude in action, a way of saying thank you for the help. There's nothing like paying gratitude forward.

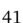

Please write notes of your thoughts about gratitude during this month. Choose an Adjective or a Phrase to describe how you feel about gratitude each day.

WEEK 1

- Monday

  _____

  _____

- Tuesday

  _____

  _____

- Wednesday

  _____

  _____

- Thursday

  _____

  _____

- Friday

  _____

  _____

- Saturday

  _____

  _____

- Sunday

  _____

  _____

WEEK 2

Monday

_____

_____

Tuesday

_____

_____

Wednesday

_____

_____

Thursday

_____

_____

Friday

_____

_____

Saturday

_____

_____

Sunday

_____

_____

WEEK 3

- Monday

  _____

  _____

- Tuesday

  _____

  _____

- Wednesday

  _____

  _____

- Thursday

  _____

  _____

- Friday

  _____

  _____

- Saturday

  _____

  _____

- Sunday

  _____

  _____

WEEK 4

- Monday

  _____

  _____

- Tuesday

  _____

  _____

- Wednesday

  _____

  _____

- Thursday

  _____

  _____

- Friday

  _____

  _____

- Saturday

  _____

  _____

- Sunday

  _____

  _____

MAY: TREAT YOURSELF

When was the last time you enjoyed some TLC?

Not every aspect of self-care needs to be hard work and drudgery. This month you're going to have some fun! It's time to give yourself a little pampering by indulging in some activities which will help to shape you in new and exciting ways all while still having the time of your life!

Get Out and About.

Take a walk in the neighborhood, take a road trip this weekend, or take a real vacation. The point here is to get a change of scenery. Don't have the means to get away? Take a virtual vacation. There are tons of tours you can take online which will give you a peek into someplace different.

Make Bathing an Artform.

Anyone can take a bath. But how many can explore all the infinite variety of baths there are? Grab a bath bomb. Explore various bubble baths.

Grab some scented soaps, and take a luxurious soak. Rose petals? Candles? A good book? It's all up to you. Take a different bath at least once a week to discover what you like and what you don't.

Get Furry.

Even if you don't have a pet, you can find some great ways to interact with animals this month with just a little bit of creativity. Volunteer at a shelter. visit the zoo. Pet-sit a friend's dog.

Adopt a new friend of your own. If you already have a pet, invest in some serious cuddle time. For a more interesting challenge, see if you can teach your pet a new trick this month.

Take Up Crafting.
There's nothing like creating things with your own hands. Now would be a great time to try a hobby which you find interesting. Or enroll in a class to go more in depth in a current hobby. Whatever you do, make a goal to finish at least one project before the end of the month.

Perk Up Your Surroundings.
It's time for some home renovation! No, you don't need a fortune. Do something small to make a room more personalised by adding a little flair. Visit thrift stores and estate sales, pick up a few pillows or plants the next time you're out shopping to give a room an entirely new look. Want to really make a change? It doesn't cost very much to put on a new coat of paint. A fresh color can make a room entirely new.

Make a Difference.
We all have causes we believe in, but we don't always do much to support them as we never feel like we have the time. If this is the case, now's the time to do something different. Volunteer. Get involved in a community project. Make someone else's life a little better in some way and you'll discover the joy which comes out of serving others. Imagine if everyone felt being active in the community was a treat instead of a chore!

Take Up Writing.

What better way to express yourself than in words? Start a journal. Pen a poem. If you're really ambitious, start the novel you always intended to write.

Give Yourself a Night Out.

What's the date you always wished you could go on? Now's the time! Pick out the perfect evening and spend the night indulging in all your favorite things. Watch a favorite movie. Eat at the restaurant you love but never seem to get to. For added fun, invite a friend to share this time with you.

Go Somewhere New.

Stuck in a rut? Try shopping somewhere you've never been before. Try a new restaurant. Go do that silly touristy thing in your community which you somehow never had time for.

Read Something.

Books are doorways into new ideas and ways of thinking. Take time this month to read something you wouldn't normally pick up. For some added fun, try out a biography or history journal or a novel in an entirely different genre just to see what you think.

Dream.

What's something you always wanted to do? Create a vision board for this idea. Daydream about it. Enjoy exploring this notion through visualisation. Then ask yourself what's something you can do to make this dream a reality. Act on it.

By the end of this month, hopefully you're feeling happier and more relaxed than you've felt in a long time.

Please write notes of your thoughts about selfcare during this month. Choose an Adjective or a Phrase to describe the type of TLC you have enjoyed and how felt each day.

WEEK 1

Monday

_____

_____

Tuesday

_____

_____

Wednesday

_____

_____

Thursday

_____

_____

Friday

_____

_____

Saturday

_____

_____

Sunday

_____

_____

WEEK 2

- Monday

  _____

  _____

- Tuesday

  _____

  _____

- Wednesday

  _____

  _____

- Thursday

  _____

  _____

- Friday

  _____

  _____

- Saturday

  _____

  _____

- Sunday

  _____

  _____

WEEK 3

- Monday

  _____

  _____

- Tuesday

  _____

  _____

- Wednesday

  _____

  _____

- Thursday

  _____

  _____

- Friday

  _____

  _____

- Saturday

  _____

  _____

- Sunday

  _____

  _____

WEEK 4

- Monday

  _____

  _____

- Tuesday

  _____

  _____

- Wednesday

  _____

  _____

- Thursday

  _____

  _____

- Friday

  _____

  _____

- Saturday

  _____

  _____

- Sunday

  _____

  _____

JUNE: SETTING HEALTHY BOUNDARIES

How do you ensure your energy is not drained by toxic people?

Being able to tell people "no" is one of the best ways to protect ourselves and our time, but how good are you at doing it? If you're like most people, boundaries might be a little bit foggy, especially when it comes to judging whether or not something might be an opportunity, or a waste of time.

As far as self-care goes, boundaries don't get enough attention. We tend not to realise just how much they do matter. Without good boundaries, our stress levels rise, which in turn can adversely affect our health. Boundaries can protect us in other ways. Healthy boundaries are necessary to keep us safe from toxic people, and stop us from wasting energy on what's not important.

How can we spend this next month in the pursuit of boundaries? Try these steps:

Create a List.
Knowing where you'd like better boundaries is the key. Start off the month with a list of areas where you feel like you don't have good boundaries, such as work or relationships. Next, list out some specific areas where boundaries are really causing you trouble, such as not being able to say no when your sister constantly needs someone to bail her out when she's short on cash.

Do a Check Up.

Not sure where boundaries might be an issue? Ask where you're feeling resentful, which is a sure sign your boundaries are out of whack. Add these points onto your list.

Create a Better Response.

With your list in hand, look for better ways to answer these boundary violations. Practicing to say 'no' can take time, so start small. Creating a script can help, especially when boundaries involve people you're close to. Going back to our example, what could you say instead to your sister when she calls asking for money? Knowing in advance will help you to say it when the time comes.

Practice Being Direct.

When it comes to good boundaries, hinting doesn't often work. You're going to have to say what you feel. To make this easier, get in the habit of being direct about your needs. Look for opportunities to speak up when you need something.

Check Yourself.

What are you feeling right now? When you pay attention to your feelings, it's easier to notice when you feel like your boundaries are being trampled.

Do Some Analysis.

Why are some of your boundaries' hot points, which are hard to enforce? Understanding you're apt to say yes to a coworker's demands because you're worried about how it would look to your boss allows you to step back and honestly assess whether your boss would even notice, much less care. It might be you've been agreeing to some things which would have served you better by saying no, all along.

Drop the Guilt.

If your emotions start getting the best of you, it's time to step back. Again, check yourself. Re-affirm this is a boundary you need to set. Remind yourself you're doing the right thing.

Enlist Help.

Who is your team? If you don't have one, this month would be a great time to form a network of supporters who have your back. Talk to them about the boundaries you're creating and ask for their help in maintaining them.

Remember, boundaries take time. You're going to have to keep resetting some of these on a daily basis until you and those around you get used to the idea. Once you do, though, you'll find this goes much easier.

Please write notes of your thoughts about setting healthy boundaries this month. Choose an Adjective or a Phrase to describe how you feel about saying 'No'.

WEEK 1

- Monday

  _____

  _____

- Tuesday

  _____

  _____

- Wednesday

  _____

  _____

- Thursday

  _____

  _____

- Friday

  _____

  _____

- Saturday

  _____

  _____

- Sunday

  _____

  _____

WEEK 2

- Monday

  _____
  _____

- Tuesday

  _____
  _____

- Wednesday

  _____
  _____

- Thursday

  _____
  _____

- Friday

  _____
  _____

- Saturday

  _____
  _____

- Sunday

  _____
  _____

WEEK 3

- Monday

  _____

  _____

- Tuesday

  _____

  _____

- Wednesday

  _____

  _____

- Thursday

  _____

  _____

- Friday

  _____

  _____

- Saturday

  _____

  _____

- Sunday

  _____

  _____

WEEK 4

- Monday

  _____
  _____

- Tuesday

  _____
  _____

- Wednesday

  _____
  _____

- Thursday

  _____
  _____

- Friday

  _____
  _____

- Saturday

  _____
  _____

- Sunday

  _____
  _____

JULY: GET OUTSIDE

When was the last time you spent some time connecting with and enjoying nature?

Who doesn't love to get outside? OK, maybe not everyone is a diehard outdoor fanatic. But whether or not you feel a yearning for the great outdoors, the benefit of nature is real. In fact, numerous studies have shown time spent outdoors has numerous health benefits. Consider these proven facts:

- Green spaces improve mood, and ease depression and anxiety
- Studies have shown hospital patients exposed to nature or even nature motifs healed faster than those who were not.
- Fresh air has been proven to help cognition.
- Just being around plants in the wintertime positively impacts Seasonal Affective Disorder.
- Exercise done outside is better for your body than the same exercise done indoors.

With so much benefit, it's definitely time to get your summer on by stepping outdoors. Here are some quick ideas to get you out into nature:

Take a Walk

This one comes up time and again in self-care just because it's so very good for you. For this month though, your walk outside is meant to be enjoyed. Go slow enough to take in several deep breaths of fresh air. Note your surroundings. Enjoy the feel of the wind on your face. Experience the sun on your skin (it's ok and even recommended to use sunscreen).

Play Like a Child

When was the last time you enjoyed some time on the swings? Or dug your toes in the sand? Or went wading in the pond? Today is your day to get a little childish. Go do what your 6-year-old self would have done when they were told to play outside.

Dig in the Dirt

There's so much benefit to working with plants. Getting into a gardening mindset is incredibly fulfilling on many levels. Create a container garden, or go all out and plant a vegetable garden. Whatever you do, savor the experience.

Nap

There's nothing like a day spent lying in a hammock with your eyes closed, listening to the sounds of nature. Having some time relaxing outside is really quite good for you.

Try Out a Farmer's Market

Interested in what other people have been doing outside? A farmer's market allows you to shop local, enjoy some whole foods, and meet some of your neighbors. A win-win all the way around!

Go On a Picnic

How about enjoying your meals outside for the month? A simple picnic allows you to enjoy what you just picked up at the farmer's market right where it's meant to be enjoyed. Outside!

Take Up Bike Riding

Riding your bike is great exercise and takes you into places your car can't go. There are beautiful bike paths everywhere.

Create

Build a birdhouse, a bat house, or even a home for bees. All these creatures would definitely appreciate your help as modernisation has endangered many natural habitats.

Get In the Water

Take a trip to the beach, go out boating, take a canoe down a lazy river, or just find a perfect swimming hole for the perfect outdoor adventure to keep you cool on a hot day.

Look At the Stars

End the day by looking up. There's something magical about the night sky. Wish on the stars, try to figure out the constellations or even just enjoy picking out the Milky Way. If you want to go all out, grab a telescope for some added fun in your stargazing.

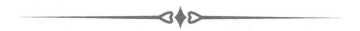

The outdoors holds too many ideas to list here, so expect to use your imagination and creativity to take you back into nature. Don't forget – nature is meant to be shared, so be sure to include those you love and show them what you enjoy most about nature too through camping and visiting the National Park system.

Please write notes of your thoughts experience about spending time outside during this month. Choose an Adjective or a Phrase to describe how you feel about spending time outside regularly.

WEEK 1

- Monday

  _____

  _____

- Tuesday

  _____

  _____

- Wednesday

  _____

  _____

- Thursday

  _____

  _____

- Friday

  _____

  _____

- Saturday

  _____

  _____

- Sunday

  _____

  _____

WEEK 2

- Monday

  _____

  _____

- Tuesday

  _____

  _____

- Wednesday

  _____

  _____

- Thursday

  _____

  _____

- Friday

  _____

  _____

- Saturday

  _____

  _____

- Sunday

  _____

  _____

WEEK 3

- Monday

_____

_____

- Tuesday

_____

_____

- Wednesday

_____

_____

- Thursday

_____

_____

- Friday

_____

_____

- Saturday

_____

_____

- Sunday

_____

_____

WEEK 4

- Monday

  _____

  _____

- Tuesday

  _____

  _____

- Wednesday

  _____

  _____

- Thursday

  _____

  _____

- Friday

  _____

  _____

- Saturday

  _____

  _____

- Sunday

  _____

  _____

AUGUST: LEARN SOMETHING NEW

As the saying goes: "You learn something every day!"

You should stop learning when you are six feet under.

How do YOU learn something every day?

We're constantly learning. Every time we pick up a book or see something new on TV our brain is making some kind of neural connection. Which is good, right?

It might be. But is it good enough? As we grow older, these kinds of connections break down. We're more at risk for problems such as dementia. It becomes harder to think, and to put our thoughts into words when we do.

We can change all this though, by the simple act of making learning intentional. This means doing more than accidently picking up the stray fact. Intentional learning has a clear goal in mind. It also does wonders for your mental health, making this a crucial component of self-care. When you're constantly learning, you think better. You protect your brain against dementia. You even feel more positive and upbeat. The act of learning can even improve your heart health, and affects your self-esteem in very positive ways. Who knew?

The nice thing? It's fairly easy to do. You pick something which interests you already, and you dive right in. Here's some quick tips for keeping the learning going:

Watch a TED Talk

Just listening to what people have to say in these inspiring talks can open your mind to new possibilities. There's thousands of TED Talks to choose from, so there's definitely something for every interest.

Learn a Life Skill

Don't know how to cook? Always wanted to learn how to change the oil in your car? Now is the time to learn. Ask someone who already is an expert to help you out by having them teach you something you always wanted to know but never learned until now.

Read Something Meaningful

Grabbing a book or magazine which teaches you something new is a quick and easy way to dive into fresh knowledge. On the go? Try an audiobook or podcast to set your brain to thinking about new things.

Play Chess

The very act of playing a complicated game will teach your brain new things every time you play. Chess is especially rewarding, as it's not hard to learn, but will keep teaching you the more you play, especially against good players.

Pick up New Words

Playing Vocabulary Games or just learning new words from the dictionary will expand your horizons in splendiferous ways.

Enjoy A New Culture

Always enjoyed Thai food but never knew the first thing about the country? Start digging into faraway places. Go online to find videos and images of unfamiliar cultures. Talk to natives. Explore history, language, and other aspects of someplace you've never been.

Have a Conversation

We learn a lot when we talk to people who think differently from us. Join a conversational group or look for people to talk to from other backgrounds, belief systems, political thought, or cultures. Ask a lot of questions, and be open-minded enough to listen to their answers, even when you don't always agree.

Take a Class

Is there something you've always wanted to learn? Now's your chance. This month, sign up for a class in something new. Learn anything from cooking to auto mechanics. Community colleges are great places to start, as are websites such as Coursera or Udemy.

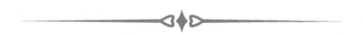

No matter what you set out to learn, so long as you're putting new information in your head, you're not doing it wrong, even if you don't become a master at what you're doing. There's a lot to be said for a smattering of new knowledge and the benefits are the same whether you earn an entirely new degree or just read interesting books on diverse topics at home. The important thing? Keeping at it, and having fun as you go.

Please write notes of your thoughts about what you have learnt during this month. Choose an Adjective or a Phrase to describe your feelings each day regarding anything you have learnt this month.

WEEK 1

- Monday

  _____

  _____

- Tuesday

  _____

  _____

- Wednesday

  _____

  _____

- Thursday

  _____

  _____

- Friday

  _____

  _____

- Saturday

  _____

  _____

- Sunday

  _____

  _____

WEEK 2

- Monday

  _____

  _____

- Tuesday

  _____

  _____

- Wednesday

  _____

  _____

- Thursday

  _____

  _____

- Friday

  _____

  _____

- Saturday

  _____

  _____

- Sunday

  _____

  _____

WEEK 3

- Monday

  _____

  _____

- Tuesday

  _____

  _____

- Wednesday

  _____

  _____

- Thursday

  _____

  _____

- Friday

  _____

  _____

- Saturday

  _____

  _____

- Sunday

  _____

  _____

WEEK 4

Monday

_____

_____

Tuesday

_____

_____

Wednesday

_____

_____

Thursday

_____

_____

Friday

_____

_____

Saturday

_____

_____

Sunday

_____

_____

SEPTEMBER: RELAX AND DE-STRESS

How are you?

Are you fine? Really? Do you feel calm, peaceful and joyful?

We all need to relax from time to time. Now more than ever, people are stressed out. We're seeing record numbers of worry and anxiety in all walks of life, especially in today's post COVID-19 pandemic. Sadly, this has a negative impact on individuals both mentally and physically. Truly, everyone needs to de-stress, and relax.

The image above demonstrates a holistic approach to relaxation and taking care of ourselves by getting together with friends and all loved ones, ideally outdoors enjoying fresh air and nature and of course good conversation, fun, and a laugh!

How does one go about telling stress to take a hike?

Reducing stress is not as difficult as you might assume. The key here is to focus on the two things which tend to work in erasing stress from your life: relaxation and using various techniques to de-stress your life to keep stress from happening in the first place.

How do we do this?

Simply Breathe

Touted as the simplest form of self-care there is, the simple act of taking several deep breaths lowers blood pressure and heart rate and helps you to relax tense muscles.

Step Back Completely

This technique is called 'grounding' and for good reason. By removing yourself from the situation, you become more grounded, and can start looking logically at what's going on instead of emotionally. Here careful analysis can be made. What exactly is the cause of the stress? How is this stressor affecting you? With this understanding, it's possible to work to remove the stressful situation, or barring that, your response to it.

Check Your Position

Your posture tells you a lot about what you're feeling. If you're stiff you're probably too tense and you might want to try a few deep breaths and some gentle movements to loosen up. Oddly enough, this will serve to relax muscles, and by extension, you. If you're slouched in, hunched over and depressed, straightening up to a more powerful stance, keeping relaxed and open in how you hold your limbs, then you'll feel more confident and ready to face challenges.

Meditate

There's been a lot of research about the effectiveness of meditation to deal with stress. Making a regular practice of mindfulness or meditation will help you to calm yourself and get back in the moment. This is especially helpful if worry and anxiety are causing the stress.

Removing Toxins

If you know what's causing the stress, it might be time to take action to remove the source entirely. Toxic people should have no place in your life. Your best option is to remove them from your life completely by refusing to spend time with them.

If this is impossible, limiting contact as much as you can will help to keep stress under control. If you're in a toxic situation (such as being in a job which sucks the life out of you) consider this your wake-up call. It's time to look for a way out.

Do the Work

A lot of stress is the result of not knowing what to do next, or feeling unsure of your skills. Taking some time to learn new things or sharpen existing skills will help to reduce this stress.

Take Some Personal Time

Don't forget to relax! If you need a personal day, and it's possible to take one, do so. Sometimes we all need a break. There's nothing wrong with taking one when you can.

Do Something You Love

Nothing drops the stress and helps you relax like getting involved in an activity which re-energises you. Plan a trip, work on a favorite hobby, or just do whatever makes you feel the most 'you.'

Try some Exercise

Many people find a great deal of relaxation in gentle exercise such as yoga or Tai Chi. Why not try a workout online or take a class to help you relax?

Turn Off Everything with a Screen

Seriously, with so much bad news in the world, the level of trolls on the internet, and the constant barrage of messages, we all need a break from time to time. Grab a timer and give yourself an hour free of electronics every day. Go read a book or take a walk outside instead.

Enjoy Being with the 'Right' People

You've removed the toxins, now head out for some socialisation with the people who'll be at your very best. Even if you only spend the time connecting virtually with positive people, you're going to see a positive impact on your mood.

No matter what you do, remember stress is always going to find you. Learning now how to handle it when it strikes will help you to cope better with the effects. Also, by setting up some solid strategies now in regards to stress, you'll be ready to shut it down the moment stress rears its ugly head.

Please write notes of your thoughts about well you have managed to relax and de-stress during this month. Choose an Adjective or a Phrase to describe how relaxed you feel each day.

WEEK 1

- Monday

_____

_____

- Tuesday

_____

_____

- Wednesday

_____

_____

- Thursday

_____

_____

- Friday

_____

_____

- Saturday

_____

_____

- Sunday

_____

_____

WEEK 2

Monday

_____

_____

Tuesday

_____

_____

Wednesday

_____

_____

Thursday

_____

_____

Friday

_____

_____

Saturday

_____

_____

Sunday

_____

_____

WEEK 3

- Monday

  _____
  _____

- Tuesday

  _____
  _____

- Wednesday

  _____
  _____

- Thursday

  _____
  _____

- Friday

  _____
  _____

- Saturday

  _____
  _____

- Sunday

  _____
  _____

WEEK 4

- Monday

  _____

  _____

- Tuesday

  _____

  _____

- Wednesday

  _____

  _____

- Thursday

  _____

  _____

- Friday

  _____

  _____

- Saturday

  _____

  _____

- Sunday

  _____

  _____

OCTOBER: HEALTHY RELATIONSHIPS

Mental health is the measure of the state of our well-being. How good are your relationships with your loved ones?

Healthy relationships are important to our well-being. But so too is the ability to practice self-care even when in a relationship. Too often we get neglectful of ourselves when we link our life to someone else, be it significant other, child, or even parent. We get so busy taking care of those around us, we forget to take care of ourselves.

Finding this healthy balance is crucial to good health. Then add to this the component where the relationship itself needs tending, and things can get complicated. Whew! It's a good thing we're taking a month out to work on this one.

What can you do?

Here are a few suggestions how to improve Your Relationships:

Establish Time Together

No relationship can thrive if you don't put the effort in to make the relationship strong between the two of you. With lovers this means regular date night. If you're a parent, schedule a game night or other fun routines which are more about playing with and connecting to your child than teaching them life skills.

Welcome Each Other Home

Everyone loves when their arrival home is celebrated. Take note of the comings and goings of people in your life. Let them know you're always happy to see them (and sad to see them go).

Learn How to Fight Properly

When disagreements happen (and they will) learn how to handle a fight properly for the sake of less frustration and stress. By sticking to "I" statements over "you" statements, and taking turns when talking, you'll get much further than you ever will in a shouting match. Good communication skills need to be practiced, which is why the next point is also important.

Have Awkward (but GOOD) Conversations

Not everything is easy to talk about, such as emotions, triggers, and honesty about how the relationship is making you feel. At the same time, these are things you really need to talk about. Learn good conversational skills. Listen a lot. Ask good questions. When it's your turn, don't hold back. Say what's on your mind in the most respectful way you know how.

Celebrate the Little Things

We all love when birthdays, anniversaries, and other important dates are remembered. In any kind of relationship, paying attention to details like these tells the other person they matter to you.

Stop Keeping Score

No relationship can survive when you hold onto grudges or bring up the past. Make a conscious effort today to forgive and forget. It's time to move on.

Do Little Things

Surprise them with breakfast in bed. Make sure the car has gas. Bring home a little treat. Small gestures tell the other person you were thinking about them today.

Get Physical

Hug. Hug often. Everyone needs physical contact. It's even been proven in studies just how damaging it is when people withhold physical contact from each other. In romantic relationships this translates to a need for a good sexual relationship as well. How to have physical contact within the challenges of physical and socially distanced boundaries? Look for other ways you can feel 'hugged' such as wrapping up in a cozy blanket while on a video chat, or even giving yourself a hug 'from them' when you're apart.

REMEMBER TO LOOK AFTER YOURSELF IN A RELATIONSHIP

SOME TIPS TO CONSIDER:

Take Care of the Physical Stuff

Are you eating regularly without skipping meals? Getting enough sleep? Remembering to exercise and practice all the other good habits you've been forming? It's easy to get so caught up in the whirlwind of a new relationship, to forget these things entirely. If you have, don't despair. Simply jump in where you are now to get back on track.

Remember Who You Are

Who were you before you were in a relationship? Hopefully you're the same person now, only better. If not, you might want to question why. Are you trying too hard to fit a certain mold? Are you holding back to keep from scaring the other person off, or to keep from hurting the relationship? If so, it's time to stop. You need to be you, regardless of who you're with. Anytime you're recreating yourself entirely just to be with someone else, it's a bad idea.

Have Outside Interests

You can't wrap up all your interests in one person. Parents are notoriously bad at this, spending so much time in the parental role they don't leave any time at all for the things which they used to love. Outside interests are necessary in any relationship. It's healthy to do things just for yourself.

Spend Time with Friends

Much like having outside interests, having other friends is also very healthy. When you shut yourself off as half of a couple or in a caregiving position, socialisation outside of those roles can disappear entirely. Here's where you might need to put in a little extra effort to stay in touch with your old friends, just to keep you connected to the outside world.

Pursue Your Own Goals

We all have things we want to do in our lives. When we're caught up with someone else, it's easy to forget these. Whether in a romantic relationship, acting as a caregiver, or just caught up in being a parent, goals seem to fall by the wayside. Remembering those goals, and making a little time to work toward them every day does wonders for your mental health, and helps to remind you your dreams have just as much value as anyone else's.

Please write notes of your thoughts about how healthy your relationships have been during this month. Choose an Adjective
or a Phrase to describe how you felt about how your relationships each day.

WEEK 1

- Monday

  _____

  _____

- Tuesday

  _____

  _____

- Wednesday

  _____

  _____

- Thursday

  _____

  _____

- Friday

  _____

  _____

- Saturday

  _____

  _____

- Sunday

  _____

  _____

WEEK 2

- Monday

  _____

  _____

- Tuesday

  _____

  _____

- Wednesday

  _____

  _____

- Thursday

  _____

  _____

- Friday

  _____

  _____

- Saturday

  _____

  _____

- Sunday

  _____

  _____

WEEK 3

- Monday

  _____

  _____

- Tuesday

  _____

  _____

- Wednesday

  _____

  _____

- Thursday

  _____

  _____

- Friday

  _____

  _____

- Saturday

  _____

  _____

- Sunday

  _____

  _____

WEEK 4

- Monday

  _____

  _____

- Tuesday

  _____

  _____

- Wednesday

  _____

  _____

- Thursday

  _____

  _____

- Friday

  _____

  _____

- Saturday

  _____

  _____

- Sunday

  _____

  _____

NOVEMBER: LIVE IN THE MOMENT
BE MORE MINDFUL

B-R-E-A-T-H-E!
Simple Be!
Let Go.
Relax.
Be Still.
Be Calm.
Be Quiet.
Focus on Being In-The-Moment.

Mindfulness has already come up a few times. Now let's dedicate an entire month to being in the moment.

Our deepest fears and worries manifest when we start thinking about the future in negative ways. Regret and depression swamp us when we get caught up in the past. This is why mindfulness is so incredibly important. Only when we're here, right in this moment can we let go and relax. When you are fully here, there is nothing to worry about and nothing to regret. You simply are.

This is a very restful state.

In terms of self-care, being able to tune into the moment is incredibly good for your health. This affects brain function, heart rate, blood pressure, and a host of other health issues. It's so good for you, even doctors are recommending time in meditation or mindfulness activities as a part of healing.

How can you be more mindful? You start with becoming familiar with the act of meditation. This is the single-most important thing to learn when it comes to mindfulness. The nice thing? You don't have to dedicate a huge portion of the day for the practice of mindfulness, nor is it complicated to learn. There are many guided practices online you can try.

The simplest form is this:

- Start with finding a comfortable position in a quiet place.

- Close your eyes and clear your mind.

- Breathe deeply. Focus on your breath. Go in through the nose and out through the mouth.

- Keep breathing. There is nothing else in the world which should have your attention. Allow your thoughts to drift and go where they will, keeping them in the now as much as possible. Keep focusing on the breathing.

- Keep doing this until you feel your body relax.

This practice, done for only five minutes every day, will create a significant change in how you feel. But if you truly want to take this to a higher level, then it's recommended you seek out some help either online or with someone who is practiced in meditation and mindfulness which can take you to the next level.

SOME THINGS TO REMEMBER:

- It's very hard to be mindful if you're not getting enough sleep.

- You absolutely must learn how to breathe correctly. Look up "Belly Breathing" and start there.

- Mindfulness can happen without meditation, simply by focusing on the moment and savoring every detail about it.

- If you find you're having difficulty concentrating, it's ok. This is a learned practice and will take time to perfect.

Please write notes of your thoughts about whether you have been mindful during this month. Choose an Adjective or a Phrase to describe how you felt about 'Simply Being' each day.

WEEK 1

- Monday

_____

_____

- Tuesday

_____

_____

- Wednesday

_____

_____

- Thursday

_____

_____

- Friday

_____

_____

- Saturday

_____

_____

- Sunday

_____

_____

WEEK 2

- Monday

  _____

  _____

- Tuesday

  _____

  _____

- Wednesday

  _____

  _____

- Thursday

  _____

  _____

- Friday

  _____

  _____

- Saturday

  _____

  _____

- Sunday

  _____

  _____

WEEK 3

- Monday

  _____
  _____

- Tuesday

  _____
  _____

- Wednesday

  _____
  _____

- Thursday

  _____
  _____

- Friday

  _____
  _____

- Saturday

  _____
  _____

- Sunday

  _____
  _____

WEEK 4

Monday

_____

_____

Tuesday

_____

_____

Wednesday

_____

_____

Thursday

_____

_____

Friday

_____

_____

Saturday

_____

_____

Sunday

_____

_____

DECEMBER: REFLECTION

Check and look at your life over the last 12 months.
Are you happy with what you see? Are you on track to achieve the goals you set for yourself for the past year? Going forward, is it time to change gears, in order to live your best life coming year?

The last month of the year is the perfect time to encourage self reflection. Part of self-care is the gentle act of assessment, to question where you are in life, and where you want to go.

This is where you check-in to see if you're still on your life's path in the way you wish to be, or whether it might be time to change course entirely.

How then do you make a practice of reflection? It's a lot easier than you might think. Start with these steps:

Set Aside Quiet Time

In order to reflect, you need to be able to gather your thoughts. You can't do this in chaos. Find a space where you can be free from distractions, where you can work through your thoughts.

Ask Lots of Questions

You need to be honestly able to assess where you are emotionally, physically, spiritually, and personally. On every level ask yourself the hard questions:

- Are you happy with your life?
- What are some areas which you feel proud of?
- What can you possibly improve?
- What feels like it's holding you back?
- What negativity are you striving to overcome?

Make a Plan

Once you have some idea of how you're doing, figure out how you want to use what you've learned. How do you want to address the problems? What changes do you need to make? What habits need to be broken still? What new habits would you like to form?

Write it Down

Reflection is good for the soul, but not if you don't remember what breakthroughs you've had. Make a practice of journaling your thoughts.

Doing It Daily

How does this translate into something you can do every day this month? Try these quick tips:

- Use every day to assess a different area of your life.
- Reflect daily by journaling about your self-care journey.
- Make a point to jot down ideas every day for what you want next year's self-care journey to look like.

Finally, do the most important thing of all: Celebrate your progress so far.
Look at all you've done! Well done, you!
Now that's the way to end a year!

Please write notes of your thoughts about the last 12 months
Choose an Adjective or a Phrase to describe how you feel about each day.

WEEK 1

- Monday

_____

_____

- Tuesday

_____

_____

- Wednesday

_____

_____

- Thursday

_____

_____

- Friday

_____

_____

- Saturday

_____

_____

- Sunday

_____

_____

WEEK 2

- Monday

  _____
  _____

- Tuesday

  _____
  _____

- Wednesday

  _____
  _____

- Thursday

  _____
  _____

- Friday

  _____
  _____

- Saturday

  _____
  _____

- Sunday

  _____
  _____

WEEK 3

- Monday

  _____

  _____

- Tuesday

  _____

  _____

- Wednesday

  _____

  _____

- Thursday

  _____

  _____

- Friday

  _____

  _____

- Saturday

  _____

  _____

- Sunday

  _____

  _____

WEEK 4

Monday

_____

_____

Tuesday

_____

_____

Wednesday

_____

_____

Thursday

_____

_____

Friday

_____

_____

Saturday

_____

_____

Sunday

_____

_____

CONCLUSION

As adults we believe in setting goals and then our focus is on achieving those goals. Goals are great, but if you want to truly enjoy your life, the goal has very little to do with how happy you will or won't be. By appreciating the journey, you can learn to find peace, happiness, and satisfaction no matter what journey you're on. It's all about focusing on the process and embracing what you already have.

This isn't to say goals aren't important. But there's so much more to be gained from the journey itself. After all, not every goal is going to be reached in your life. But you will be on some journey or another so long as you draw breath. Small steps in the right direction can turn out to be the biggest step of your life! So, take it easy, take it slow and enjoy the journey that is your life.

When we are small children, it is clear how human beings are created to be dependent on others for physical and emotional needs to be met. We need to be fed, we need to be picked up because we crave touch, love, human warmth - both emotional and physical. We all see how babies demonstrate they live in the moment, need sleep, need calm, peace and quiet. This is self-care at its very best!

Thankfully, as you've seen, it isn't difficult to embrace the journey itself and take your happiness from there. You now know the steps and have been given a handful of tips to get you started on the right foot.

It looks like it's been quite a year. As you set forth, did you remember to have fun? Sure, perhaps it's been life changing. After all, self-care is also meant to be something which eventually comes naturally.

If you've enjoyed yourself, you'll be more apt to keep up with the habits you have learnt and will have greater success. Besides, self-care should be fun. There's a lot of great tips on these pages.

Remember, the journey is certain. The rest is up to you.

At the end of your year, don't forget to keep going. These are habits meant to last a lifetime. The nice thing? Once you're aware of self-care, all of these habits will get much easier. You'll notice some changes within yourself too. You'll be healthier. Happier. Life will seem better. In fact, the next time you're asked how you are, you won't just be answering, "fine." You'll be saying you are FABULOUS! And you'll mean every word.

ABOUT THE AUTHOR

Brendah Ndebele was born in Bulawayo, the 2nd city of Rhodesia (renamed Zimbabwe in 1980), but grew up spending large chunks of her childhood staying with her elderly paternal grandmother in a remote African village with no running water, no electricity and no sanitation. Invariably, her education suffered, despite her being bright pupil and studious.

It was the household chores she was required to do, because she was a girl! When she reached secondary school level, her parents sent her to boarding school which expanded her horizons beyond the African cultural life of the 70s under colonialism.

Brendah has always loved to read from the first day she arrived in school at primary school age, one her best loved teachers, Miss Hove reported that she asked her for a book to read at home! Apparently, everyone who knew Brendah as a toddler say she would have read books earlier but for the fact that there were no books in the family home. Her mother used to read the Bible quietly in the evenings and as a child Brendah would sit and read with her mother.

Brendah's love of reading has sustained to this day. On top of the extensive reading Brendah must do as part of her business, she reads 2 books a month for pleasure!

Mr Ian D. Graham, who was a Cambridge University graduate and Brendah's English teacher at Tegwani Boarding School, encouraged her love of reading even further and gifted her several books to read. Four (4) decades on, they continue to be in touch with one another. More about that in a separate book, which Brendah is writing!

On seeing Brendah's first book about self-care, Mr Graham remarked that Brendah continues to be curious! Mr Graham also introduced Brendah to popular music by giving her very first pop record: The Beatles - Hey Jude; followed by Cat Stevens: Tea for The Tillerman. Those 2 albums remain part of her favourite and are some of her greatest treasures! Receiving those 2 records and playing them for the first time was a defining moment in her life. Brendah decided there and then that she'd come to England to study at university.

Subsequently, 4 years later she arrived at Heathrow Airport, London with just the clothes she stood up in, her passport and just a Letter of Introduction to The National Children's Home (NCH). Mr Graham had kindly arranged for her to work in one of the NCH, Children's Homes. This Charity is still in existence to this day.

Brendah went on to gain a Bachelor of Social Sciences (BA Hons) combined with Certificate of Qualification in Social Work (CQSW), a 4-year degree course, which she gained in 1980. She went on to achieve 2 Masters Degrees: an MA in Deviancy & Social Policy, which she gained in 1987; and a Master in Business Administration (MBA), which she gained in 1993, with a Distinction. What was even more remarkable was that this was way before MBAs were popular, certainly not for people working in local government. She had a stellar career in the corporate world for four decades.

Brendah is known in her circle as The Vitality Master Coach, because she turned her own life around following personal tragedy: losing both parents and all but 1 sibling within a short period of time; as well as her soulmate of her life. During this period, Brendah has also endured serious ill health: suffered from severe bronchitis every winter; coupled with pneumonia twice.

The 3rd time was when she was on her trip of a lifetime to the Far East. She was misdiagnosed there and ended close to death, but she managed to get herself on flight back to London. Brendah survived, only to be diagnosed with an Autoimmune health condition, which she has lived with for the last 12 years.

However, Brendah refused to be defined by her disability and took up power walking despite being told that she would never walk again and has completed several marathons, power walking her way round the marathon course!

Drawing from her own experience of escaping the corporate world and facing her own life-threatening health scares which severely impaired her mobility, she found the tools to bounce back with vitality, and is thriving despite living with a chronic medical condition!

Brendah is keen on sharing her strategies for success and transformative resilience with others.

She focuses on helping people to bounce back from health challenges life throws at them. Her niche is Gut Health and Burnout - specifically in irritable bowel syndrome (IBS); and the menopause.

Brendah has 40 years' experience of service development and entrepreneurial experience, she has used that knowledge to create 2 different successful businesses, one a million-pound property business.

Her approach is holistic, incorporating The Law of Attraction and creative business ideas to enable her clients to transform their life and businesses.

Brendah is an experienced keynote speaker gained from participating at numerous national events. She has been interviewed on BBC TV and Radio. She was an External Examiner for 14 years at universities all over the UK including several in the Russell Group.

Brendah is a Certified Health Coach, Certified Law of Attraction Coach, and Certified Life Coach.
Brendah is an International Best-Selling Author and also previously wrote academic books.
Brendah's passion now is self-care specifically helping busy successful people to prioritise their health as their wealth.

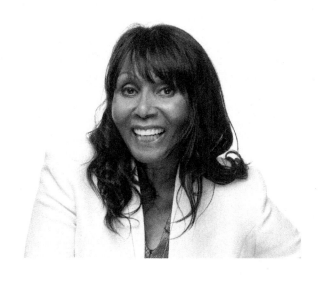

Printed in Great Britain
by Amazon

86473827R10068